Secrets to Leaner Abs

Renatta McCoy Baker

DIET

~ Diaita a way of living ~

(Greek Origin)

Exercise is the door that leads to your abs

Diet is the key that unlocks that door

Mindset controls what is allowed to enter through the door

~Coach Renatta

CONTENTS

Introduction

The Elusive Six-Pack

What is it about the abs that makes them the most coveted body part of our entire anatomy? Even if people do not aspire to a chiseled sculpted six-pack, most people want a flatter, leaner and smaller waistline. Don't you? The tummy has long been the most stubborn part of our body to transform into the abs of our dreams. For many, the abdominals are the bane of their Bikini Summer Body Goals. The saying goes "Abs are made in the kitchen" is figuratively true but we literally need more ingredients for a good ab recipe. Abs are the proverbial icing on the cake.

We 1st need an "Ab Mindset" for baking a Ab cake, figuratively speaking the mental process. After mixing all the ingredients, the cake has to bake in the oven. Now it's time to remove the cake from the oven, allow it to cool then apply the icing. The icing is the last step in baking and the presentation of your "Ab Cake". You need to develop the "Ab Mindset" for your recipe for your Six Pack Abs. The ingredients needed for an "Ab Mindset" include: A Decision, A Commitment, A Goal Plan, Execution, Determination, Consistency, Accountability, Self-Motivation and Patience.

Many believe abs are a visible sign of an ultimate healthy lifestyle, to others it's a badge of honor for the hard work and dedication put in at the gym and for some it's a complete utter vanity statement. Six pack abs will forever be the "Perception of Body Perfection". The person who has achieved washboard abs certainly has a level of respect not given to all. Whatever the reason, as to why people want the elusive six-pack abs or a tight firm waist, they want it!!! I am not here to discuss your personal reasons why but here to give you some tips on how to achieve a stronger leaner core.

Are you ready to take your abs to the next level? Well keep reading to learn more secrets to decreasing your waistline and losing a few overall pounds along the way.

Many are intimidated when it comes to achieving their ab goals. They become frustrated and doubt whether or not they will ever see the abs in their lifetime. Create the abs you want! Moreover the body you deserve by focusing on total health and wellness not just one body part. Always remember it's nice to have sculpted abs but it is much better to be in your best health to live a life of abundance. With that being said, this book will help you on your quest for abs, it will guide and assist you but you are the one who has to do the heavy lifting so if you fall off your ab goals, get back on! Going next level with your abs is going to require you learn how to master your mind in the process, your thoughts in the process and your habits in the process. Conquering your prevailing dominant "Mindset" is no walk in the park!

Eliminating all excuses, lazy habits, don't wanna do's, can't do's. Don't just read the information in this book, make it applicable to your daily habits, put the exercises to use daily, drink more water, eliminate as much stress from your life, get your required sleep, and be consistent. We all have heard of the common cast of characters that are important for ab formation such as: clean eating, cardio, cleansing, guzzling a gallon of water daily and countless crunches. Many people have set out on a journey to carve out their six pack abs and get overwhelmed and discouraged based on theory alone. It sounds too daunting to give up every food that taste good and exercise your guts out, count every single calorie you consume, worrying about the scale. All designed to drive you crazy. The journey to a chiseled six-pack is clouded with so much misinformation and a one size fits all approach that promises your results after 1,000,000 ab exercises, drinking a magical tea or wrapping your tummy like a mummy. Listen if all it took was a bunch of ab exercises to see your ab formation, I am pretty sure everybody would look like the cover of a fitness magazine. The truth is...abs require a level of commitment, discipline and work. If you do the work you will get your abs. I get this question all the time, "How long will it take me to get a six-pack"? There is no set number of days and months. It is individually based on one's personal desire and motivation and their health history. I would venture to say, if you have never worked out before and not in great shape of course it will take longer than the average person who eats pretty decent and has a habitual exercise regime.

However, individual factors such as age, your body's ability to efficiently and effectively burn fat (body type), dedication, level of commitment and consistency are the biggest key factors to seeing your ab results.

Abs in 7 days is just not a realistic goal or healthy ideal approach. Resist the diets that are too good to be true, beware of fool's gold offers that promise the abs of your dreams in 1 week. Instead aspire to the gold standard of life with healthy eating and regular exercise. There is not any one specific product or one exercise that will give you abs overnight. The truth of the matter is "Mindset is Everything!!" in achieving your ab goals. Do not allow persuasive claims that do not include healthy diet and exercise.

Chapter 1

The Anatomy of the Abdominals

The six- pack are the most recognizable ab muscles of the abdominals. They are the franchise player muscles of an entire group of muscles that make up our core. The six-pack always gets all the attention, accolades and credit. However, all of our abdominal muscles (the core) are needed for doing things that we take for granted like walking to stabilizing the thorax and the pelvis when our body is engaged in dynamic movements. Our core supports everything from our spine, posture, stability, pregnancy, pelvic floor and a healthy back. "Abs" dubbed the overall prevailing name for the midsection as if there are no other supporting muscles in this all-star lineup.

Most people only focus and train the muscles that are forward facing or the side oblique for aesthetics purposes (the look). Training your abs on a one dimensional plane will not create complete ab formation. However, training your abs for core strength, power and force produces abs of steel "The Ab Trifecta". Learning how to train your entire body will give you more opportunities to carve your mid-section into your glorious chiseled abs.

Let's take a quick look at the abdominals. Below you will find 4 distinct sections of muscle that incorporate the entire abdominal region and its corresponding function:

Rectus Abdominis: Easily recognized as the visible six-pack. These muscles count for 8 muscle bellies (used for posture and flexing lumbar spine).

Transverse Abdominis: The deepest inner layer of the abdominals not visible by sight but very important none the less (used to stabilize internal abdominal pressure).

Internal Oblique: This group of ab muscles are each located on both sides of the abdominals directly below the rectus abdominis right inside your hip bone. When twisting to the right, you are simultaneously contracting both your right and left internal oblique and your left external oblique (used to stabilize the body when conversely twisting left to right).

External Oblique: The largest set of the abdominal muscles and 2nd popular to the rectus abdominals. Your external obliques sit on both sides of your rectus abdominis. The unique function of your external obliques are twisting left and right, the opposite oblique is responsible for the stability of the body (used to stabilize the body when conversely twisting right to left).

Knowing your ab muscles and their corresponding function allows you to develop the mind muscle connection needed to transform your body. Your abs are a part of you not this external thing outside of you that you need to obtain or purchase. You already have abs now it's time to unleash your "Ab Mindset". Now that we have familiarized ourselves with our ab anatomy let's move on to the next lesson of what most influences getting that nice tight waistline.

Chapter 2

Factors that Most Influence Ab Formation

Crunches, Crunches and more Crunches.. Stop with the crunchers already! Sigh.....Why are you not seeing the results after your 1000 crunches a day challenge?

A bunch of crunches or sit-ups and every ab exercise in the book will not give you those elusive abs. If that were the case, surely, you should be a Spartan with abs or a Goddess by now if crunches were the only secret to obtaining ab formation. Don't worry all those crunches you have already done over the years are not in vein, they just will not burn the fat needed to reveal your ab formation.

The 5 Biggest Influencers of Abs

1 - **Diet:** Food Impacts everything! What are you eating? Do you eat processed and fast foods but want head turning Abs? Well the truth is that there are some people who can eat anything they want and maintain abs but most people do not fall into the flawless stellar kick butt genetics glory story. Clean eating does more for your midsection than a thousand well intended crunches. I will share the best foods for abs later in the book. But here I want to impart that if you are seriously looking to change your midsection your first goal needs to be changing your diet and the foods you eat. Cut out processed foods (manufactured foods with a shelf life) high in sugar, preservatives, fillers, sodium and unhealthy food dyes.

Cut out the white refined sugars/flour and high sucrose, fructose foods and drinks.

Read the labels know what you are consuming on a daily basis. Keep a food diary.

2 - Genetics: Let's face it genetics plays an important factor in everything down to the formation of how our ab muscles are stacked and shaped. You can crunch away all you want but it will not physically change the way your muscles are genetically made. Meaning at birth your ab muscles were created before you made your grand entrance here on earth. Genetics gives us our physical blueprint such as: our eye/hair color, height, bone structure and unfortunately, many genetic disorders. As much as our genetics are our permanent marker where we cannot change our DNA, we are still able to change and build our bodies despite our propensity towards certain unfavorable genes.

3 - **Body Fat:** Our arch nemesis! Most people worry and focus all their time and attention on a magical number on the scale known as "scale weight". We have a love/hate relationship with the scale. Scale weight takes into consideration everything from our flesh, muscles, bones, water and organs. Looking purely at the scale becomes problematic when accessing other factors that impact the condition of our body. Sure the scale tells us how much we weight at any given time and is helpful for you and doctors to provide a quick easy blush number. There are many other factors the number on the scale does not accurately reflect, which are factors such as: bone density, blood count, stress, blood sugar, and insulin levels etc.

Body Fat (adipose tissue) is necessary to store lipids from which the body creates energy. Storage fat is extra fat that forms deep in the adipose tissue known as visceral and subcutaneous.

Extra fat storage is what creates serious issues with our health. If you have large amounts of extra fat store in the adipose tissue, this is the reason you are unable to produce real ab formation.

4 - Exercise: If you have been eating properly on a consistent basis and exercising to no avail (translation: little to no ab formation or any weight loss), then it's time to take inventory of your diet and workout regimen. Contrary to popular belief long hours of cardio starts to burn your lean muscle tissue. The most efficient way to lose fat while simultaneously building lean muscle mass is to execute compound exercises that activate multiple

muscles at once. In order to do this you must perform intense muscle bearing exercises that engage your core and get your heart pumping. What I mean is you must exert force and provide resistance to tear muscle so that it will recover and rebuild itself stronger.

You don't need to exclude cardio from your routine. Cardio is needed for optimal health and aids in burning calories which results in fat loss as we know but your muscles will always need resistance to grow. Go heavier! To really see your abs you should be using the 80/20 rule. Your workout regimen should consist of 20% Cardio and 80% Resistance Strength Training.

5 - Underlying Health Issue(s): In some instances you may not be seeing your ab formation due an unknown health issue. Bloating or an enlarged stomach may not

be from over eating or lack of exercise.
There are certain illnesses that affect the
stomach and your organs in your belly. A
very common issue for women is uterine
fibroids. Many women find it difficult to
lean out around their waist due to fibroid
tumors. Other issues such as irritable
bowel syndrome and allergies to gluten and
diary will cause the stomach to swell.
Autoimmune diseases are another
underlying factor. If diet and exercise are
not effectively changing your belly bulge
you should see a doctor to identify if there
is an underlying issue.

*Disclaimer: It is important to note if you
are on any medication, your medication
may be causing weight gain. If you believe
you could be suffering from any of the
aforementioned disorders please seek the
advice from your medical doctor as to what
is the best course of action for your diet
and exercise program.

Chapter 3

The Water Vitamin Connection

The water vitamin connection is a very important factor in creating a leaner midsection. The body needs water and the proper nutrients for every cell in our body. A poor diet consisting of processed & junk foods prevents you from achieving a leaner flatter stomach. The best foods for a leaner stomach are natural "Whole Foods" that offer the highest nutritional value. **Whole foods** are foods found in nature they grow from the ground or a tree(plant based). Despite our best efforts at eating a wholesome balanced diet, we are unable to receive all of our nutrients via whole foods. In addition to eating natural whole foods you will need to supplement with a quality multivitamin to fill in the gaps.

I am sure you have heard of the term "water weight" if you have tried to lose weight around your stomach. So what exactly is water weight and why does water weight play a role in ab definition? Our bodies are made up of approximately 60 -70% water this is the normal amount of water needed for every system in our body to function properly. However, when we eat foods high in sodium and a high cholesterol diet our body's natural defense is to hold on to extra water. So water becomes trapped in our cells instead of acting as a flushing agent. Once the body retains more water than needed it adds the extra flub typically around the waist. Also, when we become dehydrated as a result of not consuming enough water our body will hold on to the water in an act of self-preservation to try and compensate for the shortage of water supply. Water weight not only adds inches to your waistline it is also reflected in scale weight.

Once you have addressed the sodium, dehydration or any other underlying problem that is producing water weight gain, you will begin to lose those first few inches or pounds relatively fast towards your abs. Drinking water is essential to life itself and needed to assist ir the development of lean muscle tone. One of the easiest ways to slim your stomach is drink plenty of water daily to flush out toxins and waste.

Mindful tips: 1 gram of carbs requires 3 to 4 grams of water in order for your body to properly process it.

Recap: Take a multivitamin and drink plenty of water.

Chapter 4

Stress Weight

Bad stress negatively impacts our entire body to include our mind, body and emotional state. Here is yet another reason to manage your stress levels as much as possible. When your body is under stress it releases a hormone in your system which has good and bad consequences. This infamous hormone is known as cortisol aka "your secret calories" that do not come from consuming food cortisol affects everything from our blood pressure down to our body's retention of water. What makes cortisol such a sneaky pesky culprit is that it can be released when you think you are eating healthy by restricting those unwanted calories and even when exercising too strenuously. Just when you think you got weight loss all figured out "cortisol" can sabotage your results.

Logically speaking, if you were cutting out those unneeded calories and exercising it should produce fat loss. However, you could possibly be activing more cortisol in your system that ultimately impacts that stomach bulge and weight gain. Stress directly affects the synchronicity of our hormones. When your stress levels are very high, it slows down thyroid functionality and throws your blood sugar levels out of range. So you are feeling good about yourself eating healthier, exercising and cutting out those midnight snacks but still noticing your weight is climbing, it could be stress causing your weight gain. Take inventory of your stress levels and make a conscious effort to eliminate your stress triggers. Do not eat when you are stressed!

10 Ways to Reduce Stress and Lower Cortisol Levels

1: Create and Focus on Positive Imagery

2: Exercise (yoga, walking, swimming)

3: Incorporate Prayer and Meditation

4: Say "No" to Unreasonable Demands

5: Be More Flexible in Achieving your Goals

6: Practice Self-Care Daily

7: Align with your True Authentic Self

8: Enjoy a Hobby and Find your Passion

9: Turn Off All your Devices

10: Accept and Embrace Change

Chapter 5

Listen to your Gut to See your Abs

This is literally the "Aha" moment you been waiting for. Here is why this phrase is so relevant when it comes to seeing your ab results. Are you bloated, feeling sluggish, extremely full, crave sweets and salty foods daily? Hmmmmmm ..... If you've answered yes to 1 or more of the above questions there is a good chance you have an over - abundance of yeast in your digestive system.

Muffin top may be a silly metaphoric way to speak about the midsection but literally most people who have problems losing weight around the belly follow a particular recipe when eating. If you are indulging in foods with high a sugar content, refined flour, diary, gluten, fatty foods versus eating a healthy well balance meal, then your dream abs in reality is a muffin top.

Did you know our bodies desperately seek to normalize the body's alkalinity? Examine the foods you're eating. It is important you hold the foods you eat to the highest scrutiny because these foods will either be assisting you with creating the abs you want or assisting you with creating the muffin top you despise. Once you identify your bad food choices start to examine your eating habits. Are you really hungry or just arbitrarily eating? Do you fill in the gaps during the day with food? Most people unconsciously eat on autopilot without really being hungry (mindless eating). Are you constantly snacking on junk food because you have given yourself easy access? Do you often crave something sweet or salty after each meal?

Do you reach for that bag of chips to read a book or watch your favorite television show? Food is a part of our social construct. We freely accept we must eat to pass the time or eat when we plain ole feel like it. The aforementioned unconscious habits are sabotaging your body goals. Let's get back to the subject of our digestive system.

There is a very good chance your digestive system and colon has an over growth of yeast. Yeast is great for baking muffin tops not good for lean trim abs. The yeast factor is real! Yeast by nature is a normal part of our digestive system. A poor diet and an abundance of sugar creates an out of balance digestive environment. Yeast prevents the body from absorbing the healthy nutrients that keep our bodies in particular the stomach lean and trim. If you notice you are still hungry after a meal and have sweet cravings your stomach's pH needs to be restored back to normal. Once your pH is restored back and healthy your digestive tract will function properly making it more conducive in seeing your abs. Inflammation in the gut prevents our body's ability to breakdown food. When the body is unable to break down food it creates inflammation in our bodies with negative side effects. The body responds to inflammation in the gut negatively with gas, irritable bowel syndrome, bloating, upset stomach and constipation.

Taking inventory of what you are eating is much more impactful than 1000 crunches or a waist trainer. Doing crunches will not create abs if the bad bacteria in your gut out numbers the good bacteria. Wearing a waist trainer will not create 6-pack abs. Clean up your diet and you will see significant improvement around your waistline.

Chapter 6

Your Digestive Gym

Unlock your ab formation with fiber rich foods. Many will opt out of real strategies and habits that produce abs and fall for claims of a six-pack overnight. There are so many products that promote rapid weight loss and abs in 7 days. There is no tummy tamer, melt belt, gut buster, flab to ab, hour glass waist in 7 days. The fat around your midsection was not created in 7 days so forgive yourself for neglecting your health and do the work! Waist trainers are everywhere promising you six-pack abs. Do yourself a favor (save your time and money) throw away all the unrealistic expectations of getting results from a fad or magical product. It would stand to reason if you place some form of binding contraption or tourniquet around your waist for long periods of time it can temporarily change the shape of your body. Essentially you will notice some localized indention and some loss in water weight. Spot training is not beneficial in real fat loss.

The specific area where the pressure is applied and forcing the body to compress will not create abs. Once the waist trainer is removed the body will adjust back to its normal shape in a matter of time. Nothing beats the benefits of plain old fiber for waist training. Our bodies require both insoluble and soluble fiber. Feeding your body the food that was designed to keep the body functioning healthy is the path way to ultimate total health. People who tend to eat foods high in fiber are leaner, less likely to gain weight over their lifetime and healthier. Your vitality and longevity depend on healthy a healthy gut.

Soluble Fiber is food that attracts water to form a gel in our digestive tract to break down food for easier removal. Soluble fiber foods are: nuts, carrots, yams, avocados, flaxseeds, sweet potatoes, beets, mangos and oatmeal to name a few. Soluble fiber interferes with the absorption of bad fat and sugar for this reason it lowers cholesterol levels in our system. Insoluble Fiber is opposite of soluble fiber in the sense it does not break down as it passes through the digestive tract. Insoluble fiber adds bulk to stools and acts as an inside scrubber to remove waste and toxins left in the colon. Insoluble fiber foods are: wheat bran, veggies, whole grains. The following foods are good sources of insoluble fiber: Coco powder, linseed, peanuts, coconut flakes, dried carrots, peas, and rye flakes. Get Moving Literally!! On your way to a six-pack naturally with fiber.

Chapter 7

"AB"solute Foods

1 *Apples*: Apples are an excellent food source for abs. The fact that Apples already contain about 80%-85% water helps satiate you into feeling fuller. In addition, apples are a very good source of insoluble fiber. Think an "Apple a day keeps the Fat away"!

2 *Salmon:* A wonderful source of Ab protein that included the good fatty acids. We normally don't want anything fatty associated with our mid- section. However, fatty acids promote slow digestion which combats spikes in glucose levels and curbs cravings.

3 *Eggs:* Many people either have converted or in the process of converting over to a meatless, non-animal consuming diet. If this is you, great for you! However, if you ever decide to change your mind or have not restricted your lifestyle to exclude all animal protein eggs are a sure bet for leaner abs. Eggs contain a substance called "choline" that boosts your metabolism. Eggs have a bad reputation for causing high cholesterol. Egg whites have found their place at the table. A good egg omelet could be your game changer in your quest for ultimate abs. Fill it with veggies and fruit on the side to be a buff chickadee.

4 *Bananas:* Wow who would have thought that getting caught with a banana in the tailpipe would be a great way to improve your ab formation. Bananas fight the good fight. Bananas are high in potassium helps minimize Belly Bloat!

5 *Quinoa*: I know you are wondering how to pronounce quinoa (Keen-Wah). A grain that that can mask itself as a baby's name. This amazing superfood grain is double the protein of many fortified breakfast cereals. How about it is 5 grams of fiber on top of 11 grams of protein not too shabby aey? Adding quinoa is a easy quick way to add fiber to your diet.

6 *Cherries*: If life is a bowl of cherries I suggest you eat cherries until your heart is content. Cherries deep dark color makes them a powerful superfood with phytonutrients and antioxidants. Shhhhhsh listen closely! It is believed that cherries actually have the ability to alter fat cells. Don't tell anyone I told you, its classified secret information that has been hidden in plain sight.

7 Tuna Fish: Not Sorry Charlie! Tuna is excellent for weight loss especially the waistline. At first blush chicken and beef come to mind when thinking high protein. Fish many times gets overlooked and dismissed when it comes to protein. Fish can be considered the strongest in the sea. Omega fatty acids are known to reduce stubborn fat cells (belly fat).

8 Almonds: Oh Almond Joy! The best thing about almonds, they are the most convenient fast way to add a quick protein boost to your diet without turning on the stove or even blending up a shake. Almonds fight off food cravings and builds lean muscle. Nuts are good way to add those essential fatty acids omega 3's.

9 Peanut Butter: A favorite food staple in my kitchen. Peanuts are chalked full of powerful protein. Do not overdo it with the peanut butter. The really good thing is one scoop a full table spoon will do the job.

10 *Grapes:* You heard it through the Grape Vine that grapes contain a very high amount of phytonutrients and anthocyanins that provide protection against free radicals. Grapes are also known for resveratrol that work against fat forming cells around our stomach.

11 *Green Tea:* So many reasons to love tea, this is worth all the tea in China. Green tea is categorized as a thermo-genetic meaning its properties increases the body's temperature to burn fat(boost your metabolism). So how much green tea do you need to drink? The answer is... you will need to consume 3 to 4 cups on a daily basis to start reaping the benefits to see your abs.

12 *Cinnamon:* Cinnamon spice can help combat insulin response in the body, stopping you from storing fat in the cells. We all wish the health benefit of cinnamon included cinnamon buns but just like carrot cake and sweet potato pie unless it is a vegan dish the desert version does not offer any health benefits. So get spicy and add cinnamon to your favorite cereal or shake!

13 *Cheddar:* A good source of conjugated linoleic acid (CLA), which helps to lose weight and build muscle. Add some cheese to a veggie omelet and maximize your breakfast. *Note: Vegan alternative take a conjugated linoleic acid supplement orally.

Chapter 8

Cardio .vs. Weights

This age old debate has been the boxing match that plays out in the gym of popular opinion and belief that one has to be better than the other at losing weight. In this corner we have "Cardio" which has long been touted as the clear winner at burning fat for years. However, in the opposing corner we have "Strength Training" or "Resistance Training", in my most humble professional opinion strength training wins the fight against deep stubborn fat. Lifting weights alone will improve your body but adding the cardio aspect to weight is most ideal for losing and maintaining a leaner body. I do not believe the debate between Cardio .vs. Weights will end any time soon so for all practical reasons and for the sake of producing ab formation, I am going on the record to say both cardio and strength training are needed for abs to show out. The most effective training method for abs is interval training which incorporates cardio in short burst and strength training with either body weight or hand held weights. Interval training is where cardio and weights no longer take an adversarial relationship. It now forms a powerful duo to provide longer lasting fat burning benefits which results in lean muscle and weight loss.

Rev up your metabolism with High-Intensity- Interval –Training (H-I-I-T) instead of the age old 60 minute treadmill workout. Once the body becomes well-adjusted to a certain level of exercise it is no longer challenged. The body will adjust and get accustomed to it. The common term is "Plateau". The body gets just as bored as if you were watching grass grow or paint dry. You want to ensure your body is constantly adjusting to new levels of growth. Changing your workout routine frequently is the difference between seeing some results versus seeing the best results for your hard earned efforts.

One little unknown secret is that the cortisol (bad stress hormone) naturally kicks in after hours of intense workouts or long drawn out cardio sessions. Yes, there is a defined art to building nice lean muscle and not losing muscle to long over extended cardio sessions or lifting. To achieve your ab goals you will have to do both cardio as well as strength training. This becomes even more of a necessity as we age. It is a fact more weight bearing exercises are needed to offset the natural progression of losing muscle mass as we grow older with time. Cross training the core is more beneficial than burn out from long extended cardio sessions.

Explosive exercising in addition to weight bearing exercises provides you with a higher and longer "After Burn Effect", after your workout is complete. The after burn effect is your body's ability to continue to burn fat long after you are finished working out. The most effective exercises continue to burn calories hours after training. Plain old cardio burns calories in the gym only versus performing resistance training that has a fat burning zone long after you have left the gym and your exercise has finished.

Chapter 9

Macronutrients or Micronutrients

Try repeating Macro-Micro 5 times as fast as you can. Getting healthy should not make you feel like you need a Master's degree in nutrition or becoming a dietician. Some terms and concepts when broken down will make more sense making it easier to apply to your healthy eating.

Understanding and knowing how the body functions and what the body requires to thrive will not only help you with improving your overall health, it will move you 10 steps closer to those long anticipated abs. You may have heard the terms "Macro" Nutrients and "Micro" nutrients and thought this jargon only really applies to serious body builders or professional athletes. Everybody could benefit from knowing what Macronutrients and Micronutrients are and how they impact our body's composition. Macronutrients are the foods that provide our bodies with calories for energy. These macronutrients come in the form of: **Protein, Carbs and Fats.** Micronutrients are other nutrients in the form of vitamins and minerals required for our body to sustain life. The terms prefix "Macro" and "Micro" in of itself refers to the amount of nutrients the body needs where our bodies require larger amount of macronutrients. Micronutrients consist of water soluble vitamins, fat soluble vitamins, trace minerals and macro minerals. Diets that restrict certain Macro or Micro nutrients can wreak havoc on the body. Eating a variety of healthy foods to include all macros and micros will create change in your ab formation. Speak to a dietician or nutritionist.

Chapter 10

Best Ab Training Method

I am often asked "What is the best exercise or best diet to get Abs of Steel? Be careful when throwing around the word "Best". The best anything is what works best for you. The word "Best" is relative to what works for your body type and personal history. I like to replace "Best" with "Most Ideal" this way it allows you to be open and flexible to tweak and personalize it as you see fit which yields your best results.

Creating great ab formation is a result of strengthening your core muscles. You will never see your abs if you do not work on getting them strong and lean. Body fat plays the bigger factor in ab formation which of course is lowered by exercise or as I prefer to say conditioning. Here is why crunches are not the best exercise to see your abs. The truth is crunches do not burn off the top layers of fat covering your abdominals. Crunches are actually great for toning and shaping once you have successfully addressed your body fat percentage. The absolute hands down most effective exercise for training your abs are explosive full body exercise that work your entire body. Specific exercises such as bodyweight: (using only your body weight) such as squats, pushups, pull ups, lunges, mountain climbers, jumping jacks, jump squats, sprints, planks, jump rope and burpees etc. The best routine(s) to gain more strength, power and balance to tighten your core section is to pe-form these body weight exercises in short burst in the form of a High Intensity Interval Training routine (H-I-I-T).

There is no real benefit to performing extended cardio sessions and long workouts to lose body fat.

As I mentioned previously, once the body has reached its maximum stress level via the stress from the load of your workout, your body starts to go in a catabolic state.

So the best training routine for your abs are short burst exercise that maximizes the body's response to resistance and force being exerted on the body.

I would like to share with you: 10 universal body weight exercises that condition your entire body in particular your core muscles using your own body weight.

What I love the most about the simplicity of natural body weight exercises is just that "It's Simple" no weights or drive to the gym required. However, it's the most natural way to enhance your natural body build and achieve a nice proportioned body. A very small percentage of humans fall into the genetic bingo of an elite athlete with Spartan abs and a body fat percentage between "2% –10%" however, body weight exercise gives the body a more proportioned appearance, slimmer waist and toned extremities.

1) **Jumping Jacks**: A tried and true Calisthenic exercise that gets the whole body moving, the energy used to jump while simultaneously vigorously swinging the arms up and downward movement is effective in raising the heart rate as well as good abduction and abduction of toning the legs and arms. Jumping jacks great full body exercise that flattens the stomach.

2) **Squat(s)**: The squat is extremely effective for building the entire body and strong core. The legs are

the largest muscle group in the body, train the biggest muscle group and your entire body reaps the benefits. Why are squats great for building ab formation? Firstly, the whole entire body is used is used to stabilize itself when squatting and you must keep your core tight and posture upright which enacts maximum tension on your core muscles. No Weights Squat (Repeat 5 sets of 25) Add Weights (Repeat 5 sets of 15).

3) **Hanging Leg Raises:** If you are serious in your pursuit of a six-pack then this exercise is the one for you. Position yourself on a bar and allow your body to freely hang. Use your core to raise your legs upward, while holding your core firm and bracing your arms and back.

This exercise not only works your core muscles it simultaneously works your opposite corresponding back muscles. Many people neglect exercising and strengthening their back muscles which are needed to build a strong all around tight core. You will not find a person who has those coveted six pack abs without those coveted back muscles.

4) **Planks:** Planks may look easy at 1st blush. However, planks are known to be brutal and effective in building a strong core. By far one of the best exercises due to its many variations to improve your whole entire body. What makes planks one of the superior body weight exercise is that it effectively strengthens your core while your arms, shoulders, neck, biceps and

legs are engaged providing maximum body coverage. Do you want to lose some of that arm fat? Planking requires the arms to absorb pressure of holding your body weight making it a great exercise to also tone your arms. Planks are a full over all bang for your buck exercise.

5) **Alternating Scissors Kicks:** This exercise targets those pesky lower abs which can be the most challenging when trying to slim down your waistline. Lay on your back, place hands underneath your hip bone. Slightly raise your legs, open and close feet one over top the other in alternating cycle (Repeat 5 sets for 30sec-60 sec).

6) **Bicycle Elbow Crunch:** The area
that provides the hour to the glass
shape figure are the oblique
muscles. Bicycle elbow crunches
are great for targeting those love
handles. Lay flat on the floor.
Hands behind neck. Raise both
legs off the floor, bring your torso
forward towards your knees,
tighten your core and guide and
extend your elbow towards the
opposite knee while alternating the
legs in and out. (Repeat 5 sets for
20 reps).

7) **Burpees:** Start off in a standing
positon with your feet positioned
shoulder-width apart. Bend knees
in so that your body is in a full
squat position with your hands flat

on floor in front of you. While squatting low, kick your feet back into a pushup with your hands open palm firmly on the ground. Lower your chest towards ground into a push up, kick your feet back towards your arms with hands open palm firmly on ground back into squatting position. While kneeling in squat position jump and propel your entire body upward with your raising your hands over your head for explosive momentum.

Beginner: (Repeat 5 sets for 5 reps). **Moderate:** (Repeat 5 sets for 10 reps). **Expert:** (Repeat 5 sets for 20 reps).

8) Abdominal Hold: (Chair Required) Sit at the edge of the

chair place hands beside your hips and thighs, palm the edge of the chair with a firm grip (ensure you are stable to prevent chair from sliding and falling off the chair), tighten your core while raising your feet 2-4 inches off the floor lift your butt off the chair and hold as long as possible. A great way to get some inconspicuous ab work in while at the office. (Repeat 10 sets).

9) **Stability Ball Rollout:** Kneel down on floor with stability ball in front of you, forward lean on ball with both forearms/elbows. Keep your back straight and your abs engaged, extend your arms out by rolling the ball as far away from

your body as possible (hold in this extended position for 5 secs), slowly roll back to starting positon. (Repeat 5 sets for 20 reps)

10) **Raised Arms Partial Sit up:** Lie flat on your back, with knees bent at 90 degrees, raise your arms shoulder length apart straight up in air. Pull your upper body half way up and hold for 10 secs and slowly return to starting position on floor. (5 sets of 15 reps)

11) **Up Hill/Inclined Sprints:** Run as fast as you can uphill and jog slowing down hill (Repeat 10 times or at your discretion and/or ability)

12) **Mountain Climbers:** Get into a straight arm plank position on hands and knees, mount both hands

shoulder distance apart, hold arms straight (do not lock your elbows), raise knees towards chest in alternate kicks. Tighten core, keep back straight do not compromise proper form. If you notice your form is slipping Stop!!, Take a breath and readjust. Build your power and pace. (Repeat 5 sets for 20 alternating kicks)

13) **Superman Swimmers:** Lay on stomach, stretch arms out in front of you in a superman position with both legs and arms 1" off the floor. Alternate hands and feet to simulate swimming. Focus on keeping your core tight. (Repeat 5 sets for 60 secs).

14) The 1 - 2 Boxing Punch Twist:

Assume a boxing stance position bring your right foot back, bring both hands up, left arm up out in front of left foot and right arm lowered in front of right foot (standing at an angle), use your left hand to punch while twisting your torso in towards the direction of the punch, bring left arm back to starting position, twist your body in the opposite direction with right punch. Left hand is 1 and Right Hand is 2. (Repeat 10 sets for 20 reps).

15) **Russian Twist:** This intense core-strengthening exercise will engage all of your core muscles. When you're in a seated position on the floor, plant raise both feet off the floor bend knees slightly. Lean slightly back, keeping your back straight and place your arms in front of you, clasp hands in front of your stomach. Engage your core and slowly twist your entire torso to the left alternate inhale and twist your entire torso to the right. (Repeat 5 sets for 20 reps).

Chapter 11

Sleep the Silent "S" in Abs

Sleep is the underappreciated hard working Cinderella that never gets an invite to the Fitness ball. The last thing anyone thinks about is sleeping when it comes to ab training. Many have the notion that sleeping translates to a lazy unmotivated out of shape person. Everything is relative within context. However, sleeping was gifted to us to reset, restore, rejuvenate and keep our bodies responsive to the daily rigors of living. If you are constantly running out of steam and getting hit with major energy zappers throughout day, your quality or lack of could be the root cause. We commonly dismiss fatigue as working too hard, being too busy or a long day at the office. We don't stop to think about why our body is craving the sweets, junk food and salty snacks because our pleasure seeking hormones are now being triggered due to sleep deprivation. Our brain says: *"Hey we didn't get our sleep last night! Just dope me up with sugar and junk food to give us some Johnny on the spot energy"*. It's pretty hard to resist the self-seeking urges of our mind when we do not get our proper amount of sleep. Sleep is very important! Power naps are quick restorative fixes sorta like being at a ¼ tank of gas and fueling up halfway but not a whole tank if you know what I mean.

The hard core truth is you can never replace your loss of sleep. It doesn't accrue or carry over to the next night. Habitual loss of sleep adds up on a cellular level over our lifetime.

Starving yourself of sleep, is only feeding your weight gain, in particular around your waistline.

Lack of sleep stresses every cell of your body and kicks in the aging process.

***Lack of sleep leading to sleep deprivation has the following serious health implications:**

> ➤ Negatively impacts our pituitary hormones
> ➤ Negatively impacts our endocrine regulation
> ➤ Negatively impacts our energy levels

The regulation of leptin, a hormone released by the fat cells that signals satiety to the brain which suppresses our appetite, is dependent on the duration of sleep. To break it down, the less sleep you get at night the fatter you get!

The Benefits of 6.5 – 8 Hours of Sleep

- ➢ Repairs Ab muscles
- ➢ Increases energy during workouts
- ➢ Faster muscle recovery & growth
- ➢ Activates protein absorption
- ➢ Fights the weight gain hormone (cortisol)
- ➢ Reduces stress levels
- ➢ Reduces hunger
- ➢ Aids in longevity and quality of life

Eat Less!

Work Out More!

Sleep More!

Repeat!

Chapter 12

Bowel Transit Time

Bowel transit times are a huge factor in seeing your ab formation. Simply put the time it takes for the food we eat to break down and digest and remove the food fully out of our system. Raw plant based foods are easily digested and travel out of our system the quickest. Cooked food, meat, processed and junk foods have the longest transit times in our body making our digestive system sluggish. The slower your bowel transit time the fuller your bowels become with waste. The average human has about 7 – 15 partially digested meals in their system waiting to be expelled. Our gut is essentially the body's sewer system to keep us healthy. If your stomach is constantly bloated your bowel transit time needs to increase. Fortunately, you can improve and speed up your bowel transit times with clean eating. Eat whole foods to include fresh veggies and fruits to increase your bowel transit times for ab muscles.

Once we become an adult our stomach remains the same size unless you opt for some reconstructive surgery to alter the size of your stomach pouch. You are able to "Reset" your internal eating thermostat. How? By eliminating certain foods from your diet, exercising and making healthy lifestyle changes resulting in changes to your internal eating thermostat. A thermostat auto regulates temperature via pre controlled conditions. Our appetite is set to a certain barometer through our habitual eating habits. If you are constantly eating the wrong foods your body will crave those foods out of habit.

Normal bowel transit times are between 12 – 24 hours after eating. Dehydration will affect bowel transit time as well ensure your water intake meets the suggested daily requirement. Many people struggle with constipation from not only the types of foods they consume but not drinking enough water to soften and move stools effectively during bowel movements. If your food is passing too quickly through your body, your body will not be able to retrieve the nutrients. If this is the case there could be an underlying issue that needs to be discussed with your doctor.

Consistently eating clean will change your eating thermostat for optimal bowel transit times.

Chapter 13

Waist Trimming Hacks

Spot reducing is not an exact science therefore you can't predict with certainty which area of the body will lose fat first. However, this does not mean we can't show special attention to a particular area of the body. The mid-section is ore of the most loathed parts of the body that equally both men and women desperately want to transform. As previously stated full body work outs in addition to cardio is highly effective to lose belly fat. Will you lose back fat or stomach fat or fat on you glutes first? The body equally distributes weight loss based on your whole entire body not just one area hence the inability to spot reduce. Before you notice the scale changing you will notice a difference in the way you feel and the way your clothes fit those non scale victories . So instead of worrying how to get rid of fat in one particular part of your body, embrace the mindset change that needs to happen. Understand your body's fat to lean ratio body composition is going through a metamorphosis that does not happen overnight.

<u>Top 10 Natural Waist Trainers</u>

1: Implement a Cleansing Regimen: Keeping your digestive tract healthy and promoting alkalinity will not only keep the bloat to a minimum it will flush away toxins that become trapped underneath the skin. ***Cleansing Teas:*** *(Ginger, Green, Red Clover, Burdock Root, Chicory, Dandelion, Fenugreek).*

2: Increase your Lean Protein Intake: Consume clean and lean sources of protein. Natural wholefoods work best.

Protein: (Tuna, Salmon, Lentils, Shrimp, Oatmeal, Avocados, Nuts, Chicken, Halibut, Eggs, Quinoa and Tofu).

3: Lift Heavier and Incorporate Bodyweight Exercises: Building lean muscle is an ageless skin tightening secret. Do not be afraid to cut the cardio short and replace with weight bearing exercises. As you build muscle all over your abs will start to shape up.

4: Cut out Sugar and Salt: Your sweet tooth may have another side that is not so sweet after all. Sugar cravings are a result of an unhealthy gut. Our gut which includes our intestines is a delicate balance of friendly bacteria and bad bacteria. **Gut health is very important!! As we consume more sugar, processed foods, salts, starches it robs our gut from absorbing the required nutrients. The magic happens, when you cut the sugar and sodium. Get ready for the disappearing act resulting in fat loss around your waistline.

5: Eat a Hearty Healthy Breakfast Daily: Get those stomach muscles pumping early and often with lean protein at the start of your day. The digestive process has a built in ab machine. Rev up your metabolism by breaking the fast of sleep with a good breakfast will keep your abs tight on the inside.

6: Develop an Eating Curfew: Get your calories in during the day and cut out all solid foods by 8:00 pm. The digestive process takes about 45 minutes you don't want to slow down or even stop the process with sleep. If the body goes into sleep mode before the digestion process is completed, undigested food gets trapped in the gut. When food is not properly digested the stomach is not emptied leaving waste behind that creates bad bacteria. So give your gut a rest before your entire body goes to sleep.

7: Perfect Your Posture: Posture is so important for the entire body in particular our core. Our abdominal muscles are important for our core as well as our spine. Engaging our core when we are sitting, standing and while exercising is another automatic way to shape your abs. Always be mindful of good posture. Head up! Shoulders back, envision an imaginary string pulling you up from the top of your head and engaged those core muscles.

8: Drink More Water: There shouldn't be a person alive that does not know that water is essential to life and a life saver to everything that lives. Even our Abs!! Especially our Abs! Drink more water to release water weight. Every cell in our body needs water. If you are not getting enough water your body will hold water deep in the cells known as "water weight". Many people don't recognize the signs when their body is in a dehydrated state. Dehydration will cause the body to retain water just like eating a diet high in sodium. You absolutely need to drink more water to nourish as well as flush your cells so the body will release unwanted water weight to reveal your abs.

9: **Intermittent Fasting:** Fasting has been around since the age of time. Fasting can be beneficial in complimenting a good workout regimen to burn fat. Give your gut a break and fast a few days every month to help manage your body fat levels. Our bodies fast naturally overnight during the sleep process where our cells are going through cell renewal. Fasting during the day is different than our nightly circadian fasting clock. During the sleep cycle our body is in the automatic rest phase we don't need fuel while the body heals and repairs. Fasting during the day requires the proper timing and quality foods to keep your energy stores above average.

*Disclaimer: Fasting does not mean starving your body of required nutrients. Fasting is a method of allowing your body adequate rest between breaking down foods in the body.

10: Take a Probiotic: Probiotics are superfoods to assist in your gut's defense against harmful bacteria. The fight against the belly bloat where your opponents are everywhere (processed foods, sugars, sodium, hormones, dehydration, stress and medication), requires some extra help from your superhero friends. A probiotic can improve your digestive eco system and strengthen the body's immune system. Add probiotics to your diet with fermented foods or a probiotic supplement.

Chapter 14

Eat Carbs and Fats!!!

While working out, your muscles use your glycogen stores for fuel. After you have finished working out, your muscles try to restore the glycogen you have depleted to rebuild muscle. Protein has long been crowned the king of muscle building. Protein is to muscle as water is to a seed that has been planted to grow. Protein is commonly promoted for workouts and to build muscle before and after but not so much carbs & fats.

Carbs and fats are feared without understanding these two macronutrients have a good and bad twin. The first thing people seek to do is restrict their diet of all carbs and fats.

Carbs and fats have become the whipping boy in this whole fight against weight gain/loss.

There are two types of carbs and fats the ones you should eat and the ones you should stay away from. Eat good carbs and fats post workout to assist with muscle recovery and growth.

Eat non starchy high fiber slow releasing carbs that provide the body with slow and steady energy for hours after eating.

Eat these foods: (sweet potatoes, oatmeal, brown rice, whole grain pasta, asparagus, bell peppers, zucchini and spinach). The word fat in of itself is offensive to many people because nobody wants to be FAT! There is a difference between Good fat versus Bad fat. Let's call the good fat PHAT: "Pretty Healthy and Tasteful".

It's time to change the perception that all fat will kill you.

Good fat is designed to keep you alive and healthy. Also if you are confused about how to differentiate good fat from bad fat here is a quick once over without being too complicated.

- ❖ *Bad Fat*: (oils that are solid at room temperature and void of any nutritional content). Known as Trans Fat ~ common food sources of trans fat include: (processed foods like chips and crackers, french fries and baked foods with hydrogenated oil).
- ❖ *Good Fat*: (polyunsaturated and monounsaturated): oils that are liquid at room temperature (olive oil, avocado oil, high-oleic safflower and sunflower oils).

Chapter 15

No Surgery Abs

Let's be honest we all have put on a few extra pounds in our lifetime. Our skin is a large organ that is heavily impacted by our weight gain and loss. Our skin has one of the toughest jobs of our anatomy in protecting our entire body and continually regenerating new skin cells to keep us healthy. When we gain weight our skin has to stretch to accommodate our growing body. Just as our skin is getting used to its new shape and size, we up and lose weight, then we gain and lose again. Our skin adjusts back and forth like a rubber band until it eventually gets stretched out of shape permanently. The skin produces extra cells when we gain weight, after weight loss the extra skin sticks around.

Weight loss is not the only reason the skin loses its elasticity. Age and gravity are constant factors and why our skin will sag and loose tightness and elasticity over time

10 Tips to Help Improve Saggy Loose Skin

1: *Exercise:*

Exercising is pretty much a cure all non-evasive skin toning and tightening technique. Exercising increase blood flow and builds tight lean muscle.

2: *Dry Brushing In a Circular Motion:*

Proper blood circulation ensures even skin tone, nutrient delivery to skin cells and healthy detoxification that ultimately tightens the skin.

3: *Apply Oils Rich in Vitamins:*

Oils are just as essential for healthy firm skin as moisture. Always apply moisture to your stomach! In addition, apply oils to penetrate and seal in moisture to assist with healing and rejuvenating the skin on your stomach: (*rosehip oil, carrot oil, mustard oil, olive oil, coconut oil, sweet almond oil, avocado oil, vitamin e oil*).

4: *Eat Foods Rich in Vitamin C:*

Vitamin C: helps to rebuild collagen. We all know citrus fruits are cleansing agents for the body. Applying Vitamin C topically can help with healing and rebuilding stretched out skin. Eat the following fruits: (*strawberries, kiwi, guava, melons, oranges, tomatoes, bell peppers, papayas and cherries*).

5: *Apply Collagen Topically:*

Our skin absorbs up to 70% of the ingredients applied to the skin. A great strategy is to apply collagen and take a collagen supplement orally.

Chapter 16

Cortisol

The Good ~ The Bad ~ The Necessary

If you are not new to health and fitness, I'm sure you have heard of cortisol by now. Many may know about or have used corticosteroids (synthetic version of cortisol used to manage and treat pain, inflammation and stiffness such as arthritis). However, cortisol is our natural steroid hormone produced by our adrenal glands. We commonly refer to cortisol as the "**Stress Hormone**" but we need a healthy balance of cortisol in order for our bodies to function properly.

Cortisol is needed in so many of our
body's functions:

- Controls blood sugar levels
- Regulates and supports metabolism
- Supports cognitive brain functions
- Supports the development of the fetus during pregnancy
- Controls our body salt to water ratio

The bad cortisol is when our body is under duress a state of fight or flight because of fear, stress or low blood sugar and releases the hormone cortisol into our bloodstream. Continuously stressing out will trigger your body's cortisol and send fat to the adipose tissue which surrounds the belly better known as subcutaneous belly fat. This fat is very difficult to shrink if you remain in a heightened stressed zone, the cortisol redeposits unused triglycerides the stubborn fat into our cells.

There are numerous reasons you should not allow stress to take over your life. Stress is often a silent killer. Learning how to manage your stress levels is important in today's society. Everybody is telling us to take the world by storm, go give it your all, don't stop, leap higher, keep pushing, max life out. Especially, when it comes to gun-ho fitness trainers, who want to push your boundaries. Trainers are telling you to hit it hard, restrict your calories, run for miles, hit the gym and after all the harsh and grueling training you still may not see your abs. Stop! Wait a minute........ Hold up! Yes we should give life everything we have and live life to the fullest. But the truth of the matter is you are creating a stressful lifestyle without rest. Abs are created with a balance of consistent diet and

exercise coupled with recovery & rest.
Slow down and breathe in the roses!
People who live very stressful lives
unconsciously tend to try fix stress and
anxiety with unhealthy lifestyle habits.
Stress accounts for 70% of doctor's visits.
Three of the biggest threats to your
lifestyle and ultimately your ab goals are:
Abusing Food, Alcohol and Smoking.
How do you relax or handle a stressful
day? Do you binge eat? Or do you feel
the need to drown your pain and stress
with alcohol or cigarettes? It is important
to recognize how you handle your
relationship with stress. If you think that
alcoholic beverage is not impacting your ab
goals think again. Alcohol has nearly twice
the calories as protein and carbs with no
nutritional value. When you consume
alcohol your body will burn it as fuel first
and postpone burning fat. Wine is more
suitable due to its benefit of resveratrol.

Chapter 17

Flabby Brain = Flabby Abs

Just that simple! If you are not exercising your mind on your health and fitness journey the greatest odds are you will never see your abs in this lifetime. Abs are a result of conditioned thoughts and repetitive habits. Your mind is your blueprint for your abs. The scale does not calculate the weight of your mind. The brain gets very little attention, it is not on display but it shows. We don't flaunt our brain in a bathing suit. Our mind is not the first thing we think about on our ab journey. No! Most people are seeking the one magical exercise or diet plan. Have you ever seen people start over and over on their health journey? They are quick to jump from product to product. Each product switch never yields any real results. Eating clean and working out is only half the real battle. The most difficult part is developing the unbreakable habits that last long enough to see real results.

Everything starts with your mental fitness. The mind needs clarity and awareness and consciousness to hit all your goals in life. **Developing a Strong Mind- Body- Soul Connection** will not only help you get "Abs" but help you keep them. Brain training includes the mental work that has to be done that creating the foundation. There will be days you want to throw in the towel because you don't feel encouraged to keep going. Your mind will constantly play tricks on you and try and revert back to your old way of thinking. You have to constantly reprogram your mind to your "New Mindset".

10 Signs You Have a Flabby Mindset

1: You only believe in a "Summer Body".

2: You look for the easy thing to do or short cuts on your health and fitness journey.

3: You think health is only aesthetic.

4: You are not interested in learning strategies and getting educated about real health for longevity.

5: You want to trade your process for instant gratification.

6: You embrace fads and overnight results.

7: You don't believe in yourself to get it done. You think your success depends on quick fixes.

8: You do not invest in mind, body, sprit and personal development.

9: You believe your results are tied to a specific product or you partake in crash diet.

10: You only want to look good and not feel good for optimal health and longevity.

If you recognize any of these as your current mindset, you will need to retrain your thoughts to get those head turning abs. Practice makes perfect. Taking action is your first step to changing your flabby mindset. Next visualize yourself being healthy and fit and how it will change the trajectory of your life. Then write down your fitness goals make it plain. Everyday work towards one or more of your fitness goals you have written down. At the end of the week track your progress and continue until you achieve your goals. Once you start hitting your goals your brain starts changing from "I Can't" to a "I Can" attitude!

Chapter 18

Meditation and Yoga

It never fails when you bring up meditation or yoga there will be a fair share of side eyes and comments "Oh the Kooky Stuff". The kooky stuff as many call it will allow you to focus and concentrate and declutter your mind to reach your ab goals. The really great thing about yoga is it has its own built in meditation which is very effective for the mind-soul-body connection. It is crucial you own your thoughts and intentions on your ab journey. Learning how to q your mind and filter out overwhelm, self-doubt, mindless thoughts and visualize your goal of six pack abs into fruition. Clearing the mind of space to create what you want makes you more aware of your daily habits.

It is our unconscious daily habits that keep us a prisoner to what we don't want versus what we say we want. Turning inward for your outward manifestation of your ab goals will kick both your mind and body to the next level.

10 Yoga Poses for Abs

Yoga poses are great for calming the mind while building your core strength. The really great thing about yoga is you can do these exercises from the comfort of your home or anywhere you desire.

1) **Boat pose - bent knee:** Come to a seated position balance on the "sit bones", place hands behind you or floor, bring feet together lift legs, bend knees (knees parallel to floor) squeeze legs together tilt slightly

back hold position (Repeat 5 sets for 20 reps).

2) **Lying Leg Reach:** Lie on your back, and raise your legs up in the air, creating a 90-degree angle with the ground. Lift your shoulders off the ground, and reach toward your left foot with your right hand. Alternate right foot with left hand (Repeat 5 sets for 20 reps).

3) **Plank with knee dip:** Start in a forearm plank position (engage core). While holding the plank, lower your right knee to the ground for a quick tap return to plank position, alternate your lower left knee to the ground for a quick tap, return to plank position (Repeat 5 sets for 20 reps).

4) **Plank Alternating Step Outs:**
Start in a plank position, hands
under your shoulders and feet next
to each other. Step your right foot
out to the side, then return to
center. Alternate with left foot out
to side. (Repeat 5 sets for 20
reps)

5) **Plank Spiderman:** Get into a plank
position with your hands shoulder-
width apart on floor. Keeping your
hips square to the floor, lift your
left leg and bring it toward your left
elbow. Return to start and repeat
with the opposite leg. (Repeat 5
sets for 10 reps)

6) **Seated Wide V Angle Straddle
Pose:** Sit on floor, legs V angle,
bring chest and pelvic forward,

keeping back flat and toes flexed.
(Repeat 5 sets for 20 reps)

7) **Hand to Forearm Plank Pose:**
Begin in a high plank position on
hands, toes tucked, elbows under
shoulders, with your core tight.
Lower your right arm to the ground
until you're resting on your forearm.
Repeat opposite side. Then, lift
back to the starting position,
alternating one arm at a time
(Repeat 5 sets for 20 reps).

8) **Downward Dog Pose:** Position
yourself on floor, press your palms
into the floor and step back with
both legs. Press your heels toward
the floor, roll your shoulders away
from your neck, and exhale. At the
end of the exhale, pull your belly
button in toward the spine. Keep

your belly pulled in as you inhale, so
that you only expand your chest.
Keep your abdominals contracted
tight and breathe deeply in and out
(Repeat 5 sets 30 secs).

9) **High Arm Chair Pose:** Position
your feet together, bend knees and
squat as if sitting in an imaginary
chair, raise arms over head (Repeat
5 sets for 30 secs).

10) **Plank Jack Pose:** Start in a plank
position, arms shoulder length apart
hands under your shoulders, bring
feet together. Jump your feet out
to a wide V, jump them back in again
(Repeat 5 sets for 10 reps).

Chapter 19

Intuitive Approach to Abs

I can't say this too many times "One Size Does Not Fit All!" So let's talk a little about realistic expectations, body comparisons and destination perfect. We often use others as our benchmark and blueprint for our goals in our lives. Especially in this day and age of social media! It's great to be inspired or admire what it takes to obtain a certain end result. However, do not fall in the trap of aspiring to look like anyone else but yourself. Expecting other people's results is like driving up to an ATM and expecting other people's money in the bank or trying to hit a moving bullseye with your eyes closed! Highly unlikely! There are many things that need to be considered such as genetics, body type, body shape, personal health history, lifestyle, diet or maybe even plastic surgery. Be sure to be realistic in your own ab goals take in consideration your age, your body type, your personal history (giving birth, thyroid disorder medications etc.). What is your body type?

> ➤ **Ectomorph:** Thin build: (Hard weight gainer hard to gain weight).
> ➤ **Mesomorph:** Athletic build: (Easy to lose weight and build lean muscle).
> ➤ **Endomorph:** Larger build: (Hard to lose weight and difficult to gain lean muscle mass).

If you are an Endomorph, do not be discouraged by your body type it simply means you have to be more conscious and make a concerted effort to make your body do what it should be doing automatically.

Your approach to getting your abs should be intuitive and personalized. Now that we got that out of the way, you can embrace your ab journey with a new resolve and new expectations that suit your personal objective and goals.

Just remember living according to other people's standards will never give you long lasting results of your own. Your resolutions to your health and fitness should be for reasons that make sense to you! Your lifestyle is personal and should be grounded in your true authentic way of living which is real true holistic health and wellness. While you may find inspiration in others and see a body type which you think is perfect, never wish for another person's body, that mindset negates your well-being and the self-confidence needed to reach your goals.

It is perfectly fine to keep healthy inspiration around you but always ensure you are working towards real results given your body, personal health history and personal goals.

Nobody has the patent on "The Best Body". It does not exist! Life does not get any better than the body you have. Own it! The best body is your body that you treat as your temple and continuously work on being the healthiest version of yourself. When you make comparisons between yourself and others, you not only give your power away you lose opportunities to love, invest your time, your energy, your resources and your focus on building a better you!

Chapter 20

Goodbye Flab ~ Hello Abs

Healthy snacks are good in keeping your body's energy levels up during the day. Most people are fighting the daily sugar blues, we grab a snack loaded with artificial sugar to give us a temporary burst of energy throughout our day.

The top 5 unhealthy food/mood addictions that are sabotaging your abs are:

- Sugar
- Salt
- Soda
- Soybean Oil
- Stress

An inordinate amount of foods claiming to be "healthy snacks" and good for you are processed foods in disguise. Beware of health foods promoting less fat and sugar, they have added fillers and additives that outweigh their health claim benefit. Also, when food is stamped "Healthy" people tend to think if they eat more and over indulge the calories won't add up. Soybean oil is found in many processed and package foods and thought to be just as harmful as sugar. Of course stress is not a food, but stress creates mood swings which triggers emotional eating (Mood Food). My recommendation is to eat tasty whole foods as snacks. The absolute best healthy snacks are raw foods that are low in calories and high in nutrients. Trade the potato chips, cookies, pastries, donuts and ice cream for superfoods and watch your abs start appearing right before your eyes.

The following are a list of great tasting superfood snacks you should incorporate into your diet:

- Almonds
- Apples
- Green/Red/Orange/Yellow Peppers
- Blueberries
- Pears
- Walnuts
- Bananas
- Grapefruit
- Pineapple
- Fruit Smoothie
- Veggie Smoothie
- Cherries
- Cucumbers
- Pumpkin Seeds
- Plant Based Protein Shake
- Whole Grain Bread/with Cinnamon
- Herbal Teas (w/honey)

Abs are a seed planted in the mind...

Cultivated and sowed in the kitchen...

Sculpted with time and dedication in the gym...

www.ingramcontent.com/pod-product-compliance
Lightning Source LLC
Chambersburg PA
CBHW061708250726
48657CB00002B/569